Psoriasis
Staying Clear

The Healthy Alternative

Leonie Mateer

Psoriasis – Staying Clear. The Healthy Alternative
Copyright © 2017 by Leonie Mateer. All rights reserved

The information in this book is based solely on the opinion and experience obtained by the author who has been a psoriasis sufferer for over twenty-five years. It is in no way meant to be a medical guide and the author advises that any change to your diet should be discussed with your medical practitioner or practiced individual.

No part of this publication may be reproduced, stored in a retrieval system or transmitted in any way by any means, electronic, mechanical, photocopy, recording or otherwise without the prior permission of the author except as provided by USA copyright law.

Published in the United States of America

1. Non Fiction: Health/Wellness
2. General Non Fiction – Health/Diet/Wellness

08/15/17
Revised: 10/07/2018

ISBN 978-0-9987014-4-8

Dedication

For all my fellow psoriasis sufferers
Looking for a healthy way to clear their psoriasis
And maintain a healthy clear skin

Foreword

There are over 125 million psoriasis sufferers worldwide. Psoriasis is a skin condition - not a disease. It is not contagious. They, the medical profession, say there is no cure but I have cleared my skin naturally – without drugs. I do know what works for me may not work for you. But there is a good chance it will – I truly hope it does.

It is important we share our knowledge and pass on our successes so all of us have the knowledge to take control of psoriasis and finally clear our skin of this embarrassing and disfiguring condition.

TABLE OF CONTENTS

Contd.... TABLE OF CONTENTS

PSORIASIS – BEFORE AND AFTER

If anyone told me two years ago that I would have clear, healthy skin after twenty-five years of embarrassment and humiliation - I would not have believed them. I had tried everything from sticky, greasy ointments, smelly tar to drugs, drugs and more drugs.

My body was covered 75% in ugly, red scales.

Living with psoriasis was humiliating, embarrassing, socially and sexually inhibiting and, if that wasn't bad enough, I was falling over with weak, sore ankles riddled with psoriatic arthritis.

And, worse, I didn't qualify for the wonder drug, Enbrel, due to MS in my family. "Too risky" my dermatologist said as he sent me off with another tube of greasy ointment.

So there I was, covered in red scales with no hope in sight. That was when I decided to do some serious research. What was causing my "flare ups"? Why were they becoming more frequent?

I read books, blogs and watched relevant movies and videos - until I found the answer. I knew what was causing my skin to flare. I knew why my body was sore and bleeding. I was acidic!

Testing my pH balance with pH test strips confirmed it. I was "off the chart" on the acidic side. *My body had been starved of alkaline foods.*

I had a purpose. I would change what I ate. I would drink alkaline water and keep away from acidic foods. I went shopping, grew a vege garden, downloaded a alkaline/acid food chart and stuck it to my fridge door, tested my pH level daily and watched my body begin to heal.

I noticed it first in my ankles. As soon as I *stopped eating sugar the pain and weakness began to subside.* *I stopped eating dairy and drinking coffee and black tea.* *I ate more greens and added herbs to everything.*

Slowly my skin healed. The plaques faded. The redness disappeared. I began to wear shorts and t-shirts and expose my new healed skin to the sun.

Once I learned that certain foods were causing my psoriasis to flare - I avoided them. I watch what I eat. Cashews cause my plaques to appear, other psoriasis sufferers find tomatoes and potatoes cause flare-up.

It is wonderful! Wonderful to be in control and feel the power of self-healing. If I can do it, so can other psoriasis sufferers. All we need is the knowledge.

THE "NO-NO" LIST OF ACIDIC FOODS!

I get asked often "What foods shouldn't I eat?" Of course, everyone is different and what foods cause my psoriasis to "flare up" may be different from what foods affect your psoriasis. However, there is a "no-no" list.

I would place "sugar" on my list. If you haven't seen the movie, "That Sugar Movie, you should! It changed my life.

As soon as I stopped eating sugar, my psoriatic arthritis in my ankles began to heal. *I used to limp and even topple over at times - my ankles were so weak. Now I can run. I haven't had a tweak of pain or weakness since.*

Giving up sugar was a major player in healing my psoriasis naturally.

The second "no-no" is dairy. Wow! Not only did I see results in my psoriasis.. *but two years later I have lost all my excess weight and have maintained a slender body for the first time in my life. Dairy was a trigger for me.*

I don't even miss it now.

Other no-no's include vinegar (replace with lemon or lime juice) black tea and coffee (replace with herbal and rooibos teas), soy sauce, mustard and meats. Oh, and alcohol.

Remember, when you start to balance your pH in your body you will start with 80% alkaline foods and 20% acidic foods. But once your skin has cleared you can go to 60% alkaline and 40% acidic.

I have my favorite acidic foods and choose them in my 40% everyday. However I have eliminated sugar and dairy completely from my diet.

If you have an acid heavy day.. drink lots and lots of alkaline water to help to balance you ph.

Many psoriasis sufferers have "food flare ups".

These can be different for everyone. I have been told that tomatoes and potatoes affect some psoriasis sufferers. They don't affect me.

However cashew nuts caused my psoriasis to flare up. Now that you are aware how foods affect your psoriasis, keep a watch on any food reactions and you will learn to avoid foods that irritate your skin.

HIMALAYAN SALT - THE ALKALINE HERO

When I decided to give up sugar and dairy to heal my psoriasis - I hoped I didn't have to give up salt too! I didn't! I learned that pink Himalayan Salt is highly alkaline and was relieved.
What a hero! I threw out all my old salts and headed for my local health food shop. It tastes amazing! And "pink" - so pretty!

I purchase both the course salt for my salt grinder and the finely ground salt for cooking and sprinkling on almost everything from radishes to sweet potato chips. Love it!

If you research this amazing salt, you will learn; Himalayan Salt benefits are quite amazing.

Containing at least 84 naturally occurring trace elements in their natural mineral form, the Benefits of natural Himalayan Crystal Salt include: Regulating the water content throughout your body and Promoting healthy pH balance in your cells, particularly your brain cells. Promoting blood sugar health.

So, not only does it help to promote healthy pH balance but has so many other benefits.

Keep a pink saltshaker in your bag or pocket

Yep. Take it with you. Keep it handy. Handy for dining out, food on the go and whenever your food needs a little alkaline fix!

HOW TO TEST YOUR PH LEVELS

I could hardly wait to test my pH levels once I heard Psoriasis grows in an acidic body. I ordered my pH test strips online but couldn't wait for them to turn up in my letterbox so I hopped into my car and drove to the nearest hardware store.

I figured the pH Test strips I had used in the past to test my hot tub water would work on me too. I was right. They worked fine. I was so acidic - I simply jumped for joy! That was the beginning of my journey to clear my psoriasis and bring back my once perfect clear, healthy skin.

Now I test my pH levels almost daily. When I see that I am slipping into the danger zone (towards the acid level - I increase my alkaline water intake and eat more alkaline foods until I am in the perfect zone 7.0 - 7.5.

So how do you do it? Well the instructions are on the package, which features a color chart You simply dip the end of the stick into your saliva. I spit some saliva into a cup and dip in the stick - it is not recommended to dip the stick into your mouth

You only need to leave it in the saliva for a second or two then take it out, and match the colors on your stick to the color chart on the package. Presto.. You have your pH level. What is it? Are you acidic?

It is not about changing you pH balance (you can't) but rather maintaining a healthy pH balance. It is not about making your pH highly alkaline 8-9-10 (you would be dead) It is all about eliminating acidic foods in order to maintain a healthy balance and, in turn, healthy skin.

Learning this simple fact changed my life. It did! Finally I could take control of my psoriasis. I had a place to start.

Two years later I have clear healthy skin. My pH levels stay at optimal levels and by being away of what I eat I can maintain my clear skin.

BAKING SODA AND PSORIASIS

My choice of ensuring my drinking water is alkaline is using baking soda (from my local health food shop). The amount needed is so small - just 1/8 tsp. of baking soda to my 8oz glass of water.

However, it is recommended to alternate your alkaline choices by switching to fresh lemon juice and/or liquid chlorophyll (derived from plants) so you are not ingesting too much baking soda long term. (Always check with your doctor before starting a new eating program).

Baking Soda (Bicarbonate) is an alkaline substance naturally produced in the body that buffers acids and helps keep pH in check.
"Many of us think of baking soda as an ingredient used for cooking, or even something that helps to keep our refrigerators odor-free, but baking soda is surprisingly good for your health and home too.

Some of the most common baking soda benefits include:

- *Eases stomach pain*
- *Helps with digestive issues*
- *Relieves bloating and gas*
- *Fights off diseases*
- *Neutralizes acid*
- *Kills fungi, mold and parasites*
- *Minimizes cough and sore throat*
- *Reduces the duration of cold and flu*
- *Helps pH balance*
- *Reduces the symptoms of gout*
- *Promotes kidney health*
- *Treats urinary tract infections*
- *Reduces muscle pain and fatigue*

British researchers found that adding one-half cup of baking soda to bathwater soothed itchiness and irritation in patients with psoriasis. I always add a soft gel capsule of evening primrose oil to my bath water also. And a paste made of baking soda mixed with a little water and dabbed on sunburn, insect bites, allergic rashes, and skin exposed to poison oak/ivy reduces discomfort. That same paste also makes a nice, gentle defoliant.

Use as a Natural Deodorant. Simply mix about a teaspoon of baking soda with enough water to create a milky liquid, and rub it on your feet and underarms. Who Knew?

Warning: Oral use is also safe, provided you do not exceed the recommended doses, as this could upset the body's acid-base balance. Larger amounts can cause temporary nausea and diarrhea.

However, the amount I am talking about (1/ 8tsp. per 8 oz. glass of drinking water and not exceeding 1/2 tsp. per day) is not excessive.

Ref: Dr Axe – baking soda
https://draxe.com/baking-soda-uses/

LEMONS, LIMES AND GRAPEFRUIT - WHO KNEW?

Welcome to the world of alkaline fruits!

I always thought these fruits were acidic... Who knew they turned alkaline in your body?

Lemons are a wonderful quick alkaline additive!

- *Squeeze lemon juice on your fish.*
- *Add a squeeze to your drinking water to boost its alkaline level to keep you pH balanced.*
- *Combine with olive oil to make an alkaline dressing for your green salads.*
- *Squeeze fresh lemon on your cauliflower before cooking to keep it white*
- *Squeeze fresh lemon juice over your guacamole (avocado mix) to keep it green*
- *Squeeze fresh lemon juice into a glass of hot water or herbal tea*

Lemons have so many health benefits Lemon is a diuretic, (assists with the production of urine) Helps with clearing toxins and bacteria, Lemon in water is calorie free and an antioxidant, Reduces the production of free radicals (anti-aging). It's antibacterial property helps fight throat infections.

I remember the days when my Mother would hand me a glass of warm water with freshly squeezed lemon when I had a cold.

Massage fresh lemon juice on your bleeding gums or toothache. (Rinse quickly if it burns) It helps stop bleeding gums and tooth pain.

For us "over 60s" it is great for lightening age spots. Just rub on area and leave for 15 minutes. Then rinse.

Flaky scalp? Massage two tablespoons of lemon juice into your scalp and rinse with water. Then stir one teaspoon of lemon juice into a cup of water and rinse your hair with it. Repeat daily while needed.

Grapefruit makes a fresh and healthy breakfast treat.

Grapefruits support clear, healthy skin

They can help to lower our risk for many diseases and conditions and may even help with weight loss as part of an overall healthy and varied diet.

The powerful nutrient combination of fibre, potassium, lycopene, vitamin C and choline in grapefruit all help to maintain a healthy heart.

The health benefits of lime include weight loss, skin care, improved digestion, relief from constipation, eye care, and treatment of scurvy, piles, peptic ulcer, respiratory disorders, gout, gums, urinary disorders, etc.

The first fruit that comes to mind in terms of medicinal uses is the reliable lime. This sour citrus fruit can do what many advanced medicines cannot. Lime, bearing the scientific name Citrus Aurantifolia, has been used for ages in the treatment of various ailments.

Add limes to your new alkaline eating program, add to avocado dips and add to water and tea. Make a ginger and lime marinade for fish with a little avocado oil

THE "NO NO" LIST OF ALCOHOLIC DRINKS FOR SKIN CONDITIONS.

I have always enjoyed a glass of champagne or a glass of wine. Champagne, to me, was a sip of celebration. Just the pop of the cork and the pouring of sparkling clear bubbles into a tall-stemmed glass made me feel a sense of excitement.

Sharing a glass of great New Zealand Sauvignon Blanc over a home cooked meal was equally rewarding.

Recently the receptionist at my dentist and I began a discussion about alcohol and skin conditions. She had suffered from a red ugly rash across her neck and upper body and had no success from doctors. Finally, in desperation, she met with a nutritionist who advised her to stop drinking wine and, in particular, red wine and champagne. She did and her rash completely disappeared.

I knew alcohol contained "no –no ingredients" but had chosen to ignore them as I had already given up so much to keep my psoriasis at bay. I decided it was time to face the affect alcohol has on skin conditions and, in my case, on psoriasis.

So, when I read 'white wine, like mixed cocktails and beer, contains sugar, in addition to some salt. Wine can lead to swollen skin and bloating,' - I was horrified.

Red wine was even worse "red wine is actually the most harmful drink for those with skin issues like rosacea- "Over 70% of rosacea sufferers had severe flare ups caused by drinking red wine!"

Oh dear. I had already eliminated sugar (so I thought) and dairy and now I was sentenced to a lifetime of zero social drinking.

I had proven sugar causes skin conditions by spiking your insulin levels, causing inflammation throughout the body. What I didn't realize was the type of sugar in alcohol was even more damaging.

I decided to look at what options I had and found a clear message on various psoriasis websites.

THE "NO NO'S OF ALCOHOLIC BEVERAGES

All red and white wines, sparkling wines, champagnes, brandy, cognac, sherry, cinzano, vermouth, port, samos, all egg and nut based liqueurs, grand marnier, and cointreau.

So what is on the "yes" list of alcoholic beverages? That is what I wanted to find out and was shocked to learn I can have a drink (in moderation) and keep my skin healthy and clear. The following list is based on my research and from websites listed as reference.

THE "YES LIST" OF ALCOHOLIC BEVERAGES

Vodka, gin, rum, and whiskey and tequila – all have 0 grams of sugar per ounce *(and zero carbs) - great options for having that occasional drink –without consuming harmful ingredients.*

But beware - most mixed drinks come packed with added sugar. So a squeeze of fresh lemon or lime, poured over ice cubes and/or a dash of water keeps it psoriasis safe.

Shots are also a great option, since there's no extra sugar, salt or other harmful ingredients.

KEEP HYDRATED – ALCOHOL IS A DIURETIC

Alcohol pulls away liquids from your body, leading to dehydration. When you have eczema, psoriasis, or any other skin disease, your body needs to stay properly hydrated in order to properly flush out toxins and to avoid inflammation
Drinking an excess amount of alcohol without properly hydrating can have a really negative effect on your skin.

I always add a small pinch of baking soda to my drinking water (even in water used for hot drinks) and drink at least 4 glasses of water a day- so if I am choosing to have a drink of alcohol, I add a couple more glasses of alkaline infused water to ensure I am keeping my body hydrated.

ALCOHOL IN MODERATION

Remember. Everything in moderation... drinking more than 1 alcoholic drink per day for women and 2 drinks for men is not recommended.

~~~~~~~~~~~~~~~~~~~~~~~~~

Alcohol and Psoriasis references:
http://www.huffingtonpost.com/2013/10/24/alcohol-skin_n_4146391.
http://www.livestrong.com/article/32276-types-hard-alcohol-sugars-carbs/
http://www.flawlessprogram.com/alcohol-causes-eczema-true-or-false/
~~~~~~~~~~~~~~~~~~~~~~~~~

PSORIASIS FOODS - WHAT HEALS!

*It should be easy, shouldn't it? Just downloading a food chart of all the perfect foods to heal your psoriasis. But it isn't that easy. Why? Because everyone is different. What foods I love, you may hate. **It is all about working out what foods from the "yes" list you can add to your everyday meals** and know you are not only healing your skin - but also enjoying every bite.*

I have spent a lifetime of dieting to lose weight - I must have lost the same thirty pounds a hundred times. It always came back. Healing your psoriasis is not about diet. It is about making your body so healthy your red, scaly body simply turns into clear, healthy skin.

And a wonderful side effect - your body weight settles at your optimum healthy level. No more yo-yo!

It is about educating you and celebrating in the knowledge that you can finally take control of this disfiguring skin condition and heal yourself forever. It is not about deprivation.

So lets talk food. I get asked, "What do you eat for

breakfast, lunch and dinner?" I find it easier to choose the foods I like from the alkaline food group and simply add them to my meals.

When my body was covered in psoriasis I ate 80% alkaline food and 20% acidic food.

I just chose the acid food I couldn't live without and added heaps of alkaline food to it.

If I want to eat eggs (acidic) I would add peppers, fresh parsley and spinach and onions (alkaline)

If I want chicken (acidic) soup I would add tons of vegetables and herbs i.e. ginger, garlic, onions, chilli pepper, sweet potato and vegetable stock and a big bunch of fresh herbs from my garden.

If I felt like Mexican food - I would eliminate the dairy (cheese, sour cream etc.) and enjoy avocado, garlic, chilli peppers, fresh lime juice, tomatoes, refried beans and corn chips.

My only rule was to totally eliminate two acidic food groups that caused psoriasis flare-ups: sugar and dairy.

I had psoriatic arthritis in my ankles. As soon as I

eliminated sugar my symptoms dissipated - all symptoms have now gone.

As a sugar junkie I thought giving up sugar would be a nightmare.

It wasn't. I have lost all cravings for sugar now. This is my third year without Easter eggs... I smile just knowing I am no longer addicted to chocolate, deserts and everything sweet.

Now my psoriasis has healed, I eat 60% alkaline foods and 40% acidic foods. If I stray my plaques begin to re appear... I drink more alkaline induced water (adding 1/8tsp of baking soda (from a health food store) or freshly squeezed lemon or lime to every glass of drinking water) and add more greens to my meals until my pH level is balanced again.

It is all about enjoying every meal and knowing you have conquered the psoriasis beast!

LET'S TALK HERBS! A PSORIASIS HEALER!

There is nothing more rewarding than picking fresh herbs from your very own herb garden.

I cut an assortment of parsley, thyme, oregano, basil, rosemary, mint and sage and tie them into a bunch with string and add it to my soups and stews.

Called a "bouquet garni" - which I remove before serving - of course.

Sauté garlic, ginger and onions in olive oil or avocado oil and add vegetables and stock - a great base for any soup or stew. Place your fresh herb bouquet on top and simmer!

Add freshly ground pepper and Himalayan salt to taste.

Add spinach or silver beet before serving for an extra alkaline burst!

Check your alkaline food chart and create your own alkaline soup. You can download a acid/alkaline food chart off the internet – there is also a chart in my book "PSORIASIS – THE SIMPLE CURE – WHO KNEW?

Add wonderful flavor and increase your alkaline intake by chopping up a fresh bunch of assorted herbs and sprinkle them generously over your meat and grilled veges before cooking.

Keep fresh hot chillies handy... finely chop and sprinkle over soups, curries, fries, eggs and grilled meats for that extra punch of "hot spice".

The Washington Post says "These luscious leaves — parsley, basil, cilantro, mint, thyme, oregano, rosemary and the like — not only add enticing aroma, fresh flavor and vivid green color to food.

Herbs have remarkable health benefits.

The true power of herbs lies in their wealth of protective polyphenols, ***plant compounds with potent antioxidant and anti-inflammatory effects.***

Piles of studies show that polyphenols in herbs help combat such diseases as cancer, heart disease, Alzheimer's, diabetes and more. Polyphenols are anti-microbial, so they can help protect us from harmful bacteria as well" And for a natural breath freshener bite into a sprig of Parsley.

Sage is an herb. The leaf is used to make medicine.

Sage is used for digestive problems, including loss of appetite, gas (flatulence), stomach pain (gastritis), diarrhea, bloating, and heartburn. It is also used for reducing overproduction of perspiration and saliva; and for depression, memory loss, and Alzheimer's disease. Wow!

Women use sage for painful menstrual periods, to correct excessive milk flow during nursing, and to reduce hot flashes during menopause.

Sage is applied directly to the skin for cold sores; gum disease (gingivitis); sore mouth, throat or tongue; and swollen, painful nasal passages.

Some people inhale sage for asthma.

Cilantro: One of my favorites and one of the World's Most Powerful "Superherbs"

Also called coriander or Chinese parsley, cilantro is both delicious and nutritious and a powerful antioxidant.

Cilantro contains vitamins A and K, as well as high levels of vitamin C and the trace mineral manganese.

Cilantro also contains an impressive line-up of other vitamins and trace minerals such as B vitamins, calcium, iron, zinc, phosphorus, potassium, and magnesium.1

- a natural preservative and has antibacterial elements.... wow!

Cilantro has long been used as a natural remedy for upset stomach, including bloating and gas, heartburn, and stomach cramps.

Add cilantro to scrambled eggs, avocado dip, soups, and salsa and as a topping on salads.

Fresh herbs add a wonderful flavour and aroma to our foods while increasing our daily alkaline food intake.

Herbs References – See Page 73

MOISTURIZE - FOR CLEAR, HEALTHY SKIN

Twenty-Five years of scaly, red, sore skin was a nightmare - to say the least! But what was even worse... dry, red, sore skin!

As my psoriasis began to heal and my skin returned to normal I knew that keeping my body moisturized was key in keeping it clear and healthy.

One of the major psoriasis "no no's" is never, never, never let your skin get dry and scaly. Daily moisturizing is essential to keep your psoriasis in check!

Many years ago I discovered a wonderful cream that is perfect - non-greasy, non-perfumed, healthy and wonderful to apply all over my body. My dermatologist, at the time, prescribed it and ever since I use it on a daily basis. A large pottle and lasts for months and months.

Non-Ionic Cream - Cetomacrogol 1000 BP

So check with your doctor first - but I highly recommend this cream for all psoriasis sufferers!

So when to moisturize? The answer is simple - daily, even twice daily! *Immediately after I bathe, I moisturize my body before it dries completely. Once your body has been exposed to the air for too long, it becomes less absorbent. So towel off and moisturize.*

Bath Time is so important for psoriasis sufferers. Medical experts say keep the water warm - not "hot" and soak in the bath for at least twenty minutes. This gives your skin time to soften. I always use a big scoop of baking (bicarb) soda, and lavender oil. Nothing like propping your laptop on a nearby stool and watching a movie or listen to your collection of relaxing music.

What if you still have plaques and dry patches?

I have used Daivonex ointment for many years. All during my psoriasis years - this cream or ointment became my "stand by".

Daivonex Ointment Calcipotriol 50 microgram/g
Applied twice daily

Again check with your dermatologist or medical practitioner - you need a prescription for this medication also.

If you have red, scaly patches - apply the Daivonex Ointment to the areas making sure you rub completely into the plaques - then apply the Non-Ionic cream to your whole body. This keeps your body moist and supple and prevents your plaques from cracking and scaling.

Having lived with psoriasis for so many years, I have tried so many products. These two products work every time.

Daivonex seems to work the best when it is fresh and from a new tube. I have tried Daivobet (with steroids) but my body reacts badly to steroids and, as a long term, option - I wouldn't recommend it.

STRESS - A PSORIASIS TRIGGER

Yep. As if stress is not bad enough on our minds and bodies ... it is worse on our psoriasis!

Just Google how stress affects our bodies and the list goes on and on.... from headaches, chest pain, fatigue to muscle tension, sleep problems and so much more...

It makes us anxious, overwhelmed, irritable, sad, depressed angry ..oh and our psoriasis flares up and bleeds and hurts and makes our stress even worse.

So what can we do? Life is tough. There is work and bills to pay and responsibilities and family to take care of.

Before my body was covered in psoriasis I would spoil myself with an hour of massage - it was heaven. All the stresses of the day would simply dissipate. Sometimes I would get a pedicure - loving the foot massage and the warm water soak. Both of these stress releases were taken from me when my skin became 75% covered in red, scaly plaques.

As for relationships - that's more stress. Covering our bodies, hiding our marked skin, lights off, feeling embarrassed - ashamed.

During the twenty-five years as a psoriasis sufferer I used food as my stress reliever... turning into a yo-yo dieter.

The more stressed I became, the fatter I became and the worse my psoriasis became.

It is all very well to say "exercise". It is a proven stress reliever... but somehow a lemon meringue pie and a good movie would win out.

It is when we are the most stressed that we must be our own best friend. Be kind to ourselves. Remind ourselves that we are not alone in our psoriasis bodies. Over 125 million psoriasis sufferers are living life with this disease. And now many of us are learning to heal our psoriasis without drugs, without all the side effects of medication. We have discovered a healthy way to eliminate the effects of this disfiguring disease. Psoriasis grows in an acidic body - it is all about learning what foods help maintain a healthy pH balance.

And, guess what? A side effect of eating the right foods transforms our bodies into the "hey, I look healthy and slender and fantastic" category!

I finally conquered psoriasis. I conquered the stress of living with this awful skin condition *by learning what foods affected my psoriasis. It gave me a purpose, a goal.*

Today I am psoriasis free. My skin is clear. My body is healthy. My weight remains the same - it doesn't fluctuate.

We can't eliminate all of life's stresses, but we can take control of our bodies.

We can get more sleep, eat less acidic foods such as sugar, dairy, coffee, black tea and alcohol and eat more herbs and vegetables and healthy avocado and olive oils and replace the junk-food salts with alkaline Himalayan salt and take walks in the sunshine and breathe fresh air and squeeze fresh lemon juice into our daily drinking water. And take regular relaxing baths with a scoop of baking soda and a soft gel capsule of evening primrose oil - your skin and mind will love it.

Somehow when we look and feel great all the other stresses seem much more manageable.

LIQUID CHLOROPHYLL - THE GREEN HEALER!

For two weeks the local shops up here in the far north of New Zealand have been out of green leafy vegetables. No lettuce, silver beet, broccoli or spinach. Stormy weather ruined the local crops (including mine) and, as the days progressed, my body began to go into withdrawal.

I found myself actually craving green leaves.

If you had told me this a couple of years ago - I would have laughed. Ice Cream, lemon pie maybe...but greens? That was before I healed my psoriasis and learned to eat foods that healed my skin rather than cause "flare-ups".

Then I remembered my liquid chlorophyll in my fridge. It is a great source of Vitamins A, C, E & K. Chlorophyll is a pigment in green plants that transfers light into energy.

For me, it is minty, tasty drink of green vegetables that helps keep me pH balanced and my skin clear of psoriasis.

The instructions are on the bottle. (5 mls. or 1 teaspoon twice daily). I like to add 1capful to my glass of drinking water and keep it chilled with ice. The drops are great when you are traveling but I prefer the chlorophyll concentrate. There is only one flavour I really like. It is a "fresh mint flavor". Some versions are rather bitter - so check out your options.

There are known side effects so check with your doctor before taking it. It's also possible that chlorophyll could negatively interact with medications you are taking.

You can make your own:

NATURAL CHLOROPHYLL

The blog Cook almost Anything shows how you can make your own liquid chlorophyll supplement by using parsley and water. Three ounces of parsley makes about 2 tablespoons of chlorophyll. You can then use your homemade chlorophyll for a tasty smoothie recipe.

Plants that are fresh and green are probably a good source of chlorophyll. This means vegetables and herbs such as:

- *Wheatgrass*
- *Green beans*

- *Spinach*
- *Parsley*
- *Arugula*
- *Peas*
- *Leeks*

One cup of raw spinach contains about 24 milligrams of chlorophyll. Parsley has about 19 milligrams per cup. You can blend parsley with water to create a "liquid chlorophyll" drink. Other greens will average 4 to 15 milligrams per cup. Your best source of chlorophyll will come from veggies and herbs that are green, inside and out. Veggies like broccoli and asparagus may be green on the outside but their whitish interior indicates a smaller amount of chlorophyll.

So, if you are not getting your fair share of greens... liquid chlorophyll is a great substitute and a pleasant icy drink as an everyday option for keeping you pH balanced and psoriasis clear!

SLEEP AND PSORIASIS

When my psoriasis flared leaving my body covered in red, bleeding sores I could always associate the flare up with lack of sleep.

Sure, my diet may have been more acid and I may not have been outside in natural sunlight recent days, but every time my psoriasis flared - I knew it was time to make sure I got good night's sleep.

Sleep is a psoriasis healer - I know.

When I awake after a great night's sleep of at least 8 to 10 hours - my psoriasis flare-up has subsided.

Did you know that while you sleep your body actually repairs and restores itself?
Here are some interesting facts:

With lack of sleep your body makes more ghrelin and less leptin. Ghrelin is a hunger hormone, and leptin is a hormone that tells you when you're full. Research indicates that people eat 300 less calories per day when they are well rested! Wow..

While you sleep your brain is sorting out what it wants to keep and what it wants to store. Try asking yourself a question before nodding off and see if the answer pops into your head when you awake. Amazing isn't it?

Getting at least 7 - 9 hours of sleep makes you happier and lessens symptoms of depression.

Sleep helps to encourage tissue growth, fight bacteria, attack viruses (you make more white blood cells when you are sleeping) and you are less likely to come down with a cold with regular, healthy sleep.

Your body eliminates toxins while you sleep and your blood pressure dips and gives your heart a rest too.

I have read that the hours before mid-night are the most productive sleeping hours - so getting to bed by 9p.m. is a good habit to get into.

There is a lot of conversation about clearing your room of electronic devices or at least turning them all OFF when you go to sleep to ensure a healthy sleep. Hard to do.. but essential for a calm sleep atmosphere.

Decades of flying for business and grabbing sleep on a plane have left me with a sleep habit. I sleep with an eye mask. It has become my "sleep trigger". As soon as I place it over my eyes - I feel myself drifting off. It also prevents me from waking to the morning light. My eyes have always been light sensitive and this simple little habit has been a great sleeping tool.

Apparently, the best position to sleep is on your back with your arms loosely by your sides and your legs slightly apart... no crossing of arms or twisting yourself into a ball (Oh dear, I do this) and let all that nice healing energy have a clear pathway to every organ of your body.

So next time your psoriasis flares - take a good "healing sleep" - turn off your iPhone, computer, television and music, put on some comfy sleepies, make sure your pillow is not too high, affix your eye mask, lay on your back, relax your body and sleep for at least nine hours.

FRUIT AND SUGAR - WHAT YOU SHOULD KNOW.

Sugar is on the list of acidic foods. Acidic foods are on the "no no" list for psoriasis sufferers. So when I read, "Which Fruits have the most sugar" on WebMD. I just had to pass it on.

Note: 4 grams of sugar - equals one teaspoon of sugar

I was excited to see that one Avocado has only a half a gram of sugar - Yeah!!!

Fruits with high sugar content:

Mango - 1 has 45 grams of sugar - Wow!

Grapes - One cup of grapes has 23 grams of sugar

Cherries - 1 cup of cherries has 18 grams of sugar

Pear - 1 medium pear has 17 grams of sugar

Watermelon - A medium wedge of watermelon has 17 grams of sugar

Figs - 2 medium size figs have 16 grams of sugar

Banana - 1 medium banana has 14 grams of sugar

Dates - 1 medium date has 16 grams of sugar

Apple - 1 medium has 19 grams of sugar

Pomegranate - 1 medium has 38 grams of sugar

Raisins (seedless) 1/2 cup has 43 grams of sugar

Fruits with low sugar content:

Guavas - one has only 5 grams of sugar and 3 grams of fiber

Raspberries - 1 cup only 5 grams of sugar and 8 grams of fiber

Cantaloupe - medium wedge only 5 grams of sugar

Papayas - half of papaya has 6 grams of sugar

Grapefruit - Half a Grapefruit has 8 grams of sugar

Lemon and Limes - Each has only 2 grams of sugar

Olives - one cup has zero grams of sugar

Plum - 1 medium has 6 grams of sugar

Kiwifruit - 1 medium has 6 grams of sugar

Avocado - 1 Avocado has 1/2 gram of sugar

Strawberries - 1 cup has only 7 grams of sugar

Other Fruits:

Apple - one apple contains 10 grams of sugar

Pineapple - 1 cup of fresh pineapple contains 14 grams of sugar

1/2 cup of canned pineapple contains 17 grams of sugar.

1 oz. of dried pineapple has 16 grams of sugar

Peach - one medium has 13 grams of sugar

Orange - 1 medium has 13 grams of sugar

Apricot - 1 cup has 15 grams of sugar

So before you pick that fruit and pop it in your mouth... choose one that helps and not hinders your path to clear, healthy skin.

TRAVELING WITH PSORIASIS

Be Prepared! Take it with you! Keep you body pH balanced throughout your day!

If you don't have fresh lime or lemon juice to add to your drinking water, use 1/8 tsp. of baking soda.

Or a few drops of liquid chlorophyll to every 8 oz. of drinking water.

Make sure you have at least 4 glasses of water throughout your day.

Before you head out the door, tuck an alkaline Himalayan saltshaker in your bag or pocket.

Bring your alkaline food with you!

I make up big pots of soups and freeze individual servings for quick access to a meal on the go.

Make you own super alkaline salad: lettuce, peppers, red onion, radish, celery, avocado with lemon and olive oil dressing.

On the Go Snacks!

Celery sticks with almond butter are a great travel snacks.
Cucumber slices chilled and sprinkled with Himalayan salt
Fresh raw radishes sprinkled with Himalayan Salt
Kale chips
Pre-cooked beetroot cut into slices and chilled
Home made salsa with corn chips
Celery and Hummus
Parsley - Fresh parsley the best ever breath freshener!!

Keep your skin moisturised!

I make sure I have a great moisturiser in my bag. Keeping your skin moisturised is key to keeping your psoriasis at bay.

My local chemist makes me up a potion - a Non-Ionic Cream. Check with your doctor or medical adviser for a recommendation. I also use a vitamin D cream, Daivonex.

Even though my plaques are now healed, I know that keeping my skin soft and moist prevents the dry patches from returning.

If you are traveling overseas, take the tiny bottle of liquid chlorophyll with you and add a few drops to your water on the plane. You cannot take fruit (lemons or limes) across borders. I sometimes travel overseas with a little baking soda in my bag. I have yet to be taken aside by customs that may question the white powder in my carry-on.

10 BEST TIPS FOR HEALING PSORIASIS

Yep. I have been there and done that - psoriasis that is. Horrible, embarrassing, emotionally and physically scarring and a relationship nightmare!

It covered my body from head to toe in long sleeved tops, long skirts and jeans. Swimming in public never happened. I stopped getting pedicures due to the disgusted stares by customers when my legs were exposed.

My body was covered 75% in red, ugly scales!

I bled in my sheets, left flakes of skin in a trail and my body was covered in slippery, greasy ointments.

That was then. This is now.
Now I am clear. After twenty-five years I have clear skin and no signs of the psoriatic arthritis in my ankles. I have been psoriasis free for two years and counting!

So I am passing on the secret to clear skin - well, it is no secret really because psoriasis sufferers worldwide (of which there are 125 million) are beginning to wake up to the fact that drugs are just concealing the effects of this skin condition - not curing it.

It wasn't until my dermatologist ran out of drug options for me that I set out on a journey to find an alternative cure.

It is the old story - we are what we eat. And if you are eating mostly acidic foods and suffer from psoriasis (like I was) then you will love how simple it is to clear your skin forever.

1. Test your pH level to see if you are acidic.

You can purchase pH test strips on line (Amazon etc.) or pop into your local hardware store. The pH test strips used for spas and pools work fine too. I check my pH level regularly to keep on track and keep my psoriasis away. The human body is supposed to be between 7.0 and 7.5.

2. Go Sugar-free

Sugar is a major reason why we suffer from so many diseases. Once humans only ate sugar when it was in season. Unfortunately it is not only "in-season" everyday now it has become an automatic additive disguised in so many of our foods. Check out "That Sugar Film" - it changed my life.

When I cut out sugar, the pain and weakness in my ankles disappeared so quickly.

3. Go Dairy Free

So easy to do. Just switch your milk for almond or coconut milk. The benefits of going dairy-free not only healed my skin, but I lost all my excess weight. Yep, I not only have lovely, healthy skin but I am trim and lean too!

4. Alkaline your Drinking Water

This should really be No. 1. You have various options to keep your body pH balanced by drinking at least four glasses a day with the addition of an alkaline booster:

(a) Add 1/8 tsp. of baking soda to your glass of drinking water.

(b) Freshly squeezed lemon or lime juice (must be fresh)
(c) Add Liquid Chlorophyll drops to your water (read my blog on Liquid Chlorophyll)
(4) Add pH drops
I like to use baking soda (bicarb of soda) mostly. It also keeps my teeth white. Don't over-do the baking soda - too much can cause side effects... Just add 1/8 tsp. to each glass and don't exceed 1/2 tsp. per day.
Interchange these options.

5. Greens, greens, greens

Yep. Grow a vege garden if you have room. Grow fresh herbs. Add herbs to everything. Eat Kale Chips instead of potato chips, Eat spinach, broccoli, and cucumber.

Make lots of soups. Watch your psoriasis heal!

6. Himalayan Salt - it's pink and on the "YES" list

Throw away all your old salts - they are acidic and called "junk food" by many. Replace with great tasting, pink Himalayan Salt. It is totally alkaline.!!!

7. Get out in the fresh air and sunshine

I am so lucky to live in both sunny California and New Zealand where the sun shines and I can lie outside and expose my skin to the healing rays of the sun (in private) Obviously I am careful to not over expose my skin. But the natural Vitamin D of the sun really helps my psoriasis. If the sun is not an option for you, I have also used Sun Bed Treatment. But make sure the tanning bed provides both UVB and UVA light. When my psoriasis flared up - a tanning bed really helped to calm my skin and during my healing process I would take regular visits to a tanning salon in Ventura.

8. Sleep

When my body was deprived from sleep my psoriasis would flare. I noticed when I got a good night's sleep; I would awake to find my plaques were not inflamed.
Sleep is so necessary for healing your skin and your body.

9. Keep your body moisturized

Now, I don't mean greasy, slippery moisturizer, but a light moisturizer that you don't even feel but you know it is keeping your skin soft, pliable and healthy.

My chemist makes me up a great moisturizer without any added nasty ingredients. Find one that works for you and use it daily. Especially when you get out of the shower or bath. Keeping your skin soft prevents those ugly dry scales from reappearing.

10. Don't STRESS!

There is no doubt in my mind that stress is a trigger for psoriasis. I know it is hard not to be stressed when your body aches with psoriatic arthritis and your skin looks like a lizard on fire but stress causes your psoriasis to flare. But one way of eliminating stress is taking control of your life. When you take control of your life it is amazing how your stress dissipates. Every day as I watched my body heal I was excited. Every day I felt "in charge" and was no longer a slave to the horrendous skin condition that had ravaged my body.

KALE CHIPS - THE PERFECT ALKALINE SNACK!

So why Kale? I could say it is because of all the wonderful health benefits (of which there are many) but really it's because it is the one salty alkaline snack we can eat as often and as much as we want. Yeah!!

It combines three alkaline foods in one:

Kale, Himalayan salt and olive oil. Isn't that just perfect!

I was a potato chip snacker...until I discovered this trick of turning this leafy green vegetable into a naughty tasting, crunchy, salty snack.

So simple to make.

Pre-set your oven to 350 f. or 175 c.

(1) Just use a scissors to cut off the curly parts of the leaves into bite size portions.

(2) Wash the kale in a colander

(3) Dry in a salad spinner (or whatever you have) Note: leaves must be very dry

(4) Dribble over olive oil and rub it in to the leaves

(5) Sparingly sprinkle over pink Himalayan Salt (don't use any other salt - other salts are highly acidic)

(6) You can get more creative at this stage and add other spices or lemon juice (another alkaline food)

(7) Bake for five minutes in the pre-heated oven

(8) Turn the tray and keep baking for another 5 minutes (until the ends begin to brown)

(9) Eat!!!

The first time I made the Kale chips I used way too much salt... I also cooked them too long. Its all trial and error... but when I figured it out - the chips were light, tasty and surprisingly yummy!

So lets get down to why Kale is called "The new beef" and "The queen of greens" and a "nutritional powerhouse" on so many websites

Basically it is low in calories, high in iron, high in fiber, high in calcium, high in vitamins, filled with powerful antioxidants and, for all of us psoriasis sufferers, it is a great anti-inflammatory food.

Best of all - it is alkaline and on every psoriasis sufferer's healing list of healing foods.

MY FAVORITE QUICK ALKALINE SNACKS

OK. So you need to eat NOW! I know that feeling. The problem is, that is when we tend to grab "no-no" foods. And we all know what they are. The trick is to have a few trusty, easy alkaline induced snacks always within reach.

When you do your weekly (or daily) shop, make sure you have these ingredients on your shopping list:

• *Yummy Almond Butter dribbled into celery sticks!*

Two ingredients on our Alkaline list which make a creamy and crunchy snack

• *Fresh celery sticks with salty Himalayan salt*

Prefer salty not sweet? This quick and easy snack satisfies the entire salty craving.

100% Alkaline! Enjoy!

• Fresh celery sticks with Hummus

Delicious, crunchy and the perfect pair of alkaline foods that make a delicious snack.

• Vege everything snack

You can't go wrong with grabbing everything in your salad fridge drawer - throw on a plate, dip them in a little Himalayan salt and turn on a great movie!

100% alkaline!

• Superfood greens in an egg omelet!

Choose your own favorite greens to add to your omelette: Spinach, Parsley, Silver beet 'and cilantro.

The rule of thumb when choosing what ingredients to add to your meal, is keep with the 60/40 rule (60% alkaline / 40% acid)

My favourite Omelet:

Silver beet - Alkaline
Parsley - Alkaline
Alkaline induced water (mixed with eggs)
Himalayan Salt - Alkaline
Eggs - Acid

Served with Rooibos Tea - Alkaline

• *Wonderful, light, crispy, salty Kale Chips*

• *Avocado Dip (Guacamole)*

One of my favorite snacks and it is 100% alkaline!!! Yeah!

My ingredients: Mix together and serve!

- *1/2 juice lemon - Alkaline)*
- *2-3 cloves garlic, minced (Alkaline)*
- *Big pinch pink Himalayan Salt (Alkaline)*
- *Small green pepper or chopped hot red pepper (my favorite) (Alkaline)*
- *3 avocados (Alkaline)*
- *1/2 cup chopped cilantro (Alkaline)*

LEEK AND SWEET POTATO SOUP

This is one of my favorite soups!

It's simple to make, but first you have to deal with the leeks. They're notoriously sandy and dirty, and very good at hiding it, so be sure to wash them well. Start by cutting off and discarding the root ends and thick dark green parts.

Cut the leeks in half lengthwise and rinse each half under cold water, pulling apart the layers to remove any grit that's tucked inside.

To make the soup, melt the butter in a large soup pot, then add the chopped leeks and garlic and cook until soft and wilted.

Next, add the sweet potatoes, stock, bay leaves, thyme, salt and pepper. Bring to a boil, then cover and simmer for 15 minutes, until potatoes are tender.

Purée the soup with a hand-held immersion blender (or in a regular blender) until smooth.

Servings: 6

Ingredients

- *3 tablespoons olive oil spread*
- *4 leeks, white and light green parts only, roughly chopped*
- *3 cloves garlic, peeled and smashed*
- *2 pounds Sweet Potatoes peeled and roughly chopped into 1/2-inchvpieces*
- *7 cups healthy vegetable broth (I make mine with lots of herbs)*
- *2 bay leaves*
- *1 sprig fresh thyme, plus more for garnish if desired*
- *1 teaspoon Himalayan salt (the alkaline salt)*
- *1/4 teaspoon ground black pepper*
- *Chives, finely chopped (optional)*

Instructions

1. *Melt olive oil spread over medium heat in a large soup pot. Add the leeks and garlic and cook, stirring regularly, until soft and wilted, about 10 minutes. Adjust the heat as necessary so as not to brown.*

2. *Add the sweet potatoes, stock, bay leaves, thyme, salt and pepper to pot and bring to a boil. Cover and turn the heat down to low. Simmer for 15 minutes, or until the sweet potatoes are very soft.*
3. *Fish out the thyme sprig and bay leaves, then purée the soup with a hand-held immersion blender until smooth. (Alternatively, use a standard blender to purée the soup in batches; see note.) Taste and adjust seasoning with salt and pepper. If soup is too thin, simmer until thickened. If it's too thick, add water or stock to thin it out. Garnish with fresh herbs if desired.*
4. *Note: If using a standard blender to purée the soup: be sure not to fill the jar more than halfway; leave the hole in the lid open and cover loosely with a dishtowel to allow the heat to escape; and pour blended soup into a clean pot.*

I always keep individual servings in my freezer for a quick alkaline meal.

Leek & Sweet potato soup: Original recipe from: Jennifer Segal - http://www.onceuponachef.com/recipes/potato-leek-soup.html
Note: I replaced potatoes with alkaline preferred sweet potatoes. and eliminated dairy from the recipe

PUMPKIN, PEAS, SPINACH SAGE RISOTTO - FOR HEALTHY SKIN

Sometimes you just have to share a recipe you find. This one was in my little local newspaper up here in the far north of New Zealand.

A wonderful hearty meal for a stormy day and easy and quick to prepare.

I removed all the dairy (cheese) and nuts to make it psoriasis safe.

It is ready in 40 minutes and serves 4-5. (I put single portions in my freezer for a quick meal)

600g pumpkin, peeled and diced 1-1.5cm (i inch cubes)
5 cups of chicken or vegetable stock
1-tablespoon butter
1/2 red onion, very finely diced then roughly chopped
1 1/2 tablespoons finely chopped sage leaves
1 1/4 cups Arborio rice
1 cup frozen peas, defrosted
2-3 handfuls of baby spinach leaves
Chilli flakes to taste (optional)

Preheat oven to 220 degrees Celsius (425 F)

Line an oven tray with baking paper.
Toss pumpkin with a drizzle of oil on prepared tray. Season with Himalayan Salt and roast for 15-20 minutes until tender. Turn once to ensure even cooking.

When pumpkin has 10 minutes cook time remaining, prepare the risotto.

Bring stock to a simmer in a small pot then remove from heat. Cover and keep warm.

Heat a good drizzle of oil in a large, heavy-based pot on medium heat.
Add butter, onion and sage and cook for 3 minutes until softened.
Add rice, stir and cook for 1 minute until rice starts to look translucent. Add one cup of warm stock and cook for about 3 minutes, stirring often, until all liquid from the first cup has been absorbed.

Repeat with one-cup measures until all stock has been added, this process will take about twenty minutes, or until rice is tender.

Halfway through adding the stock, fold peas and 2/3 of the roasted pumpkin through risotto then continue with the process of adding remaining stock.

Finely chop spinach and fold through risotto, and season to taste with Himalayan salt (Alkaline)

Divide into serving bowls and add remainder of pumpkin. Sprinkle with fresh herbs.

Note: I like to add a few chopped slices of a small red-hot chilli pepper to my recipe or I just sprinkle over chilli flakes before serving.

~~~~~~~~~~~~~~~~~~~~
~~~~~~~~~~~~~~~~~~~~

NATURAL DEODORANT – ALUMINUM FREE – PSORIASIS FRIENDLY

Oh dear! When I heard from my psoriasis buddies (Yes, I do have psoriasis buddies) that deodorants contain aluminum and that aluminum is definitely not good for psoriasis sufferers... I just had to do some research.

I read "Unlike vitamins, minerals, and trace elements, the body does not need aluminum. And aluminum is no innocent or benign participant. Aluminum accumulates in the kidneys, brain, lungs, liver and thyroid where it competes with calcium for absorption and can affect skeletal mineralization. In infants, this can slow growth."

Oh, there is more... "Aluminum-containing antiperspirants prevent toxins from being expelled by the body. " Oh and it has been linked with the onset of Alzheimer's disease and even breast cancer...but I am more concerned with adding anything to my skin that is considered "not good".

So I immediately tossed my trusty deodorant into the trash bin and headed off into town in search of a healthy alternative.

And I found a great healthy product: "Crystal Essence Roll-on Deodorant." It comes in three choices: Lavender & White Tea, Pomegranate and Fragrance Free. Hypoallergenic, no Aluminum Chlorohydrate & Paraben Free!

Brilliant!! Don't you just love it when you find that someone is on top of it all. They have already addressed this problem and created this wonderful product. USA made - but I found it on the shelf at my local chemist store here in the rural far north of New Zealand.

My favorite, the Lavender and White Tea. Smells divine. I can hardly believe it's a deodorant.

You don't have to suffer with red, scaly skin - there is a way to heal your psoriasis naturally. It takes time and keeping yourself constantly informed.

Joining a psoriasis group on Facebook or over the web - keeps you up to date with other psoriasis sufferers and what works for them. Today we are healing our skin naturally, without drugs, without costly supplements, just healthy food and knowing what triggers our skin to flare.

Happy healing.

UV LAMP FOR HEALING PSORIASIS NATURALLY.

Spending my first real winter in New Zealand for some time, I was worried my lovely clear skin would begin to form psoriasis patches in the long months ahead with little sunshine and cold days.

For me, keeping my skin in the warm natural sunshine is paramount in keeping my psoriasis at bay.

So I decided to take the plunge and purchase a hand-held UVB lamp for use at home.

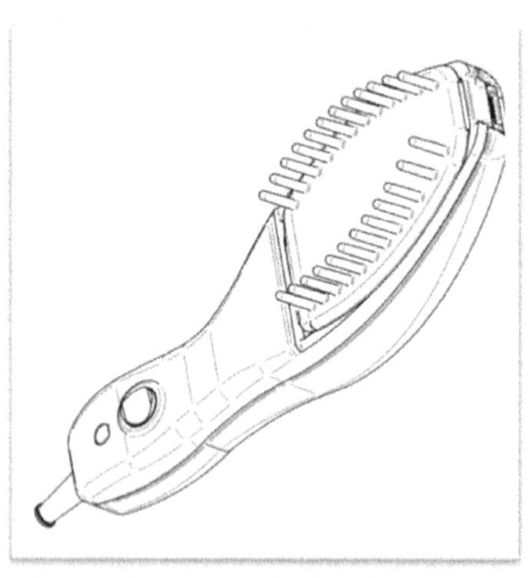

Dermfix 1000MX UV Comb

I waited excitedly for it to arrive from Australia. I wondered if it would work. (I had some little patches beginning to appear after a month without sunshine). It arrived! I read the booklet and immediately set to work - putting on the dark protective glasses, setting the little minute timer and finally switching on the lamp.

Each day for ten days I applied the light as instructed.. and presto.. it worked! Clear Skin!!

A wonderful alternative to natural sunlight. It does not feel hot on the skin - just warm.

I worked up slowly to 3 minutes per patch for the best results.. But it is important to read the instructions and use the lamp accordingly to your skin type and sensitivity to the light. It has a comb attachment which I like to use as it keeps the device at the recommended distance from the skin so I don't have to hold it in midair.

I use the timer faithfully - I turn on a favorite TV show and at the "beep beep beep" I switch to the next patch.

It is my new winter "must have". I highly recommend it.

12 BEST TIPS FOR BATHING WITH PSORIASIS

1. ***Don't bath in water too hot!***

2. Add 2 tbs. of **Baking Soda** *to alkaline the water (I purchase my Bicarbonate of Soda from a health food shop)*

3. Add a few drops of your favorite ***bath oil*** *(natural) I like lavender oil.*

4.Use a ***natural soap*** *- Aloe Vera, Oatmeal, - No fragrance.. All natural* **.**

5. Soak in water for at least twenty minutes *until all thick plaques are soft*

6. Use ***exfoliating gloves*** *to wash away flaky, loose skin.* ***Exfoliate gently*** *to avoid plaques from bleeding. It is important to remove any loose skin before you moisturize.*

7. Be careful when shaving legs (women) ***Use a razor that is flexible.***

8. Pat your skin dry with a soft towel. ***Dry thoroughly***

9. ***Immediately after drying your skin*** - *apply your Vitamin D cream to your psoriasis affected areas. (Diavonex if your Doctor has prescribed it)*

10. Apply a good non ionic **moisturizing cream** *to you whole body - fragrance free.*

11. **Bathe Daily***. It is important to keep your body soft and moisturized.*

12. **Make your bath time - your time***.* *Read a book or magazine, pop your laptop on a stool nearby and watch your favorite show, chill out and listen to your favorite relaxing music.*

HEALING PSORIASIS THE NO DRUG WAY

Greasy ointments, smelling tars, drugs that made my hair fall out, my gums bleed and my lips swell! ***Every prescription gave me hope, every drug took that away.*** *My dermatologist was at his wit's end. Finally I was approved for Enbrel! The wonder drug! But alas, MS in my family prevented me for qualifying - so there* ***I was covered 75% with ugly, embarrassing red, scales*** *and a future of covering my body from head to toe in public*

But if there is one quality I have - it is tenacity. I was determined to beat this horrible disfiguring disease - I hit the web! Research, research and research. What is psoriasis? What causes psoriasis?
What could I do to clear my skin?

When I read it - I couldn't believe it! Why, after twenty-five years of suffering with psoriasis, did I not know **psoriasis grows in an acidic body?** *This was a life-changer.*

First, I needed to find out if my body was acidic. I purchased some pH test strips from my local hardware store (for spas and pools) being much too impatient to wait for my delivery from Amazon. ***Sure enough, I was acidic!***

That set me off on a research frenzy. What foods were acidic? What could I eat? Would it work? It did - ***for three years now I have clear skin and my psoriatic arthritis in my ankles is gone!***

You truly are what you eat! Keeping my body pH balanced has enabled me to clear my skin.

As always, check with your doctor before changing your diet. My dermatologist on my last visit to him said , "You have made my day! Keep doing what you are doing."

I learned to eat more alkaline foods and avoid highly acidic foods*. I discovered what foods caused my psoriasis to "flare". I learned to keep my body alkaline throughout the day and* ***test my pH balance*** *on a regular basis.*

Today I am healthy, happy, slender and psoriasis free. One of the benefits of keeping your body pH balanced and away from highly acidic foods such as sugar and dairy is weight loss. I have always been a yo-yo dieter. ***I lost my excess weight*** *and everyday I can't believe the scales - my new weight doesn't fluctuate beyond a pound or two. What a bonus!*

Happy Healing!

ALKALINE/ACIDIC FOOD CHART

This is the food chart I use. It is from the website https://liveenergized.com - This website has wonderful tips on following an alkaline diet. - check it out!

For healing psoriasis - I ate 80% alkaline foods and 20% acidic foods until my skin healed. Then I switched to 60% alkaline and 40% acidic foods to maintain a clear skin.

I check my pH level on a regular basis to ensure that I am keeping 'Within the Zone" 7.3 - 7.5

ALKALINE/ACIDIC CHART

Highly Alkaline

pH 9.5 alkaline water (1/8 tsp. of baking (bicarb) soda in each 8oz glass of drinking water or a squeeze of fresh lemon) I purchase my baking soda from a health food store. Drink at least 4 glasses of alkaline water a day. This alkaline water was a major key to my success!!!!

Note: Do not consume more than ½ tsp. baking soda per day

Himalayan salt (Pink – either granule or fine)
(This is a must – the only salt I now use)

Grasses
Cucumber
Kale
Kelp
Spinach
Parsley
Broccoli
Sprouts (soy, alfalfa etc.)
Sea Vegetables (Kelp)
Green drinks
All Sprouted Beans/ Sprouts

Moderately Alkaline
Avocado
Beetroot
Capsicum/Pepper
Cabbage
Celery
Collard/Spring Greens
Endive
Garlic
Ginger
Green Beans
Lettuce
Mustard Greens

Okra
Onion
Radish
Red Onion
Rocket/Arugula
Tomato

Lemon
Lime

Butter Beans
Soy Beans
White Haricot Beans
Chia/Salba
Quinoa

Mildly Alkaline

Artichokes
Asparagus
Brussels Sprouts
Cauliflower
Carrot
Chives
Courgette/Zucchini
Leeks
New Baby Potatoes
Peas
Rhubarb
Swede
Watercress
Grapefruit

Coconut
Buckwheat
Quinoa
Spelt
Lentils
Tofu
Other Beans & Legumes
Goat & Almond Milk
Most Herbs & Spices
Avocado Oil
Coconut Oil
Flax Oil/ Udo's Oil

Neutral/Mildly Acidic

Black Beans
Chickpeas/Garbanzos
Kidney Beans
Seitan

Cantaloupe
Currants
Fresh Dates
Nectarine
Plum
Sweet Cherry
Watermelon

Amaranth
Millet Oats/Oatmeal
Spelt
Soybeans

Rice/Soy/Hemp Protein

Freshwater Wild Fish
Rice & Soy Milk

Brazil Nuts
Pecan Nuts
Hazel Nuts
Sunflower Oil
Grape seed Oil

Moderately Acidic

Fresh, Natural Juice
Ketchup
Mayonnaise
Butter
Apple
Apricot
Banana
Blackberry
Blueberry
Cranberry
Grapes
Mango
Mangosteen
Orange
Peach
Papaya
Pineapple
Strawberry
Brown Rice

Oats
Rye Bread
Wheat
Wholemeal Bread
Wild Rice
Wholemeal
Pasta
Ocean Fish

Highly Acidic

Alcohol
Coffee & Black Tea
Fruit Juice (Sweetened)
Cocoa
Honey
Jam
Jelly
Mustard
Miso
Rice Syrup
Soy Sauce
Vinegar
Yeast
Dried Fruit
Beef
Chicken
Eggs
Farmed Fish
Pork
Shellfish
Cheese

Dairy
Artificial Sweeteners
Syrup
Mushroom

~~~~~~~~~~~~~~~~

I hope you have enjoyed this book. If you found it helpful, I would love you to write a quick review on Amazon.

Please don't hesitate to contact me if you have any questions or want to share your own healthy natural treatment for psoriasis.

Leonie Mateer
~~~~~~~~~~~~~~~~

Leonie Mateer
ABOUT THE AUTHOR

Leonie Mateer was born and raised in New Zealand, but moved to the United States in her 30s to pursue business opportunities and now splits her time between New Zealand and the USA.

Leonie is known as the creator of the multi-million dollar TEEN brand and product line "CABOODLES".

PSORIASIS - THE SIMPLE CURE - WHO KNEW? Was her first health and wellness book followed by the sequel -**"PSORIASIS - STAYING CLEAR: THE HEALTHY ALTERNATIVE"** - a comprehensive collection of "tried and true" healthy recommendations for clearing psoriasis.

She has also written and published THE AUDREY MURDERS - a five book thriller series.

Other books include: CABOODLES - TURN YOUR IDEA INTO MILLIONS, HAVE A PRODUCT IDEA? HOW MANY COULD YOU SELL? (Business) THE MAGICAL WORLD OF DANTONIA, BLACK LAKE (Children's)

Leonie just released an online game based on her books "READ YOUR OWN FORTUNE"

Psoriasis Website: www.psoriasis-thesimplecure.com
Author website: www.leoniemateer.com

BOOK ONE

"Psoriasis – The Simple Cure – Who Knew?

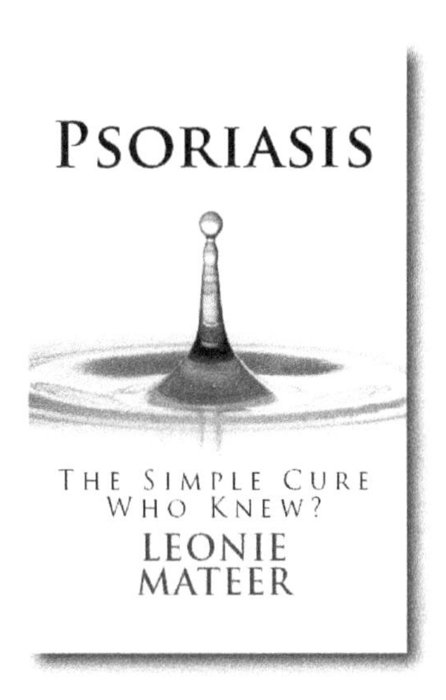

Leonie Mateer tells her story with honesty and stark humility. Living with a socially and personally disfiguring disease, she offers her readers twenty-five years of research into how to eliminate the effects of plaque psoriasis.

She tells of tried and tested cures from crystals, coal tar and ointments, to almost every drug available. She finally finds the cure in the most unexpected place.

A must read for any psoriasis sufferer.

This book also contains an Acidic/Alkaline Food Chart

References:

Dr Axe – baking soda
https://draxe.com/baking-soda-uses/

That Sugar Film
http://thatsugarfilm.com/film/watch-now/

Leek & Sweet potato soup: Original recipe from: Jennifer Segal - http://www.onceuponachef.com/recipes/potato-leek-soup.html
Note: I replaced potatoes with alkaline preferred sweet potatoes. and eliminated dairy from the recipe

Alcohol and Psoriasis references:
http://www.huffingtonpost.com/2013/10/24/alcohol-skin_n_4146391.
http://www.livestrong.com/article/32276-types-hard-alcohol-sugars-carbs/
http://www.flawlessprogram.com/alcohol-causes-eczema-true-or-false/

Making Chlorophyll
http://cookalmostanything.blogspot.com/2007/05/making-chlorophyll.html

Herbs
https://thetruthaboutcancer.com/cilantro-health-benefits/?utm_campaign=cilantro-health-benefits&utm_medium=email&utm_source=maropost&utm_content=2017-04-27&utm_term=

https://thetruthaboutcancer.com/healthy-herbs-spices/

Dermfix 1000MX UVB Phototherapy Device
Website: **https://www.dermfix.com.au/**

The Dermfix 1000MX UVB handheld lamp is a unique UVB home phototherapy device providing highly effective treatment of Psoriasis, Vitiligo and Atopic Eczema anywhere on the body. The unit is fitted with a specially developed narrowband UVB 311nm tube as standard. This model has a choice of lenses - and so can be used with or without a comb attachment.

The use of narrow-band UV-B light at around the 311nm wavelength has been well proven in many clinical trials for the treatment of many common skin conditions.

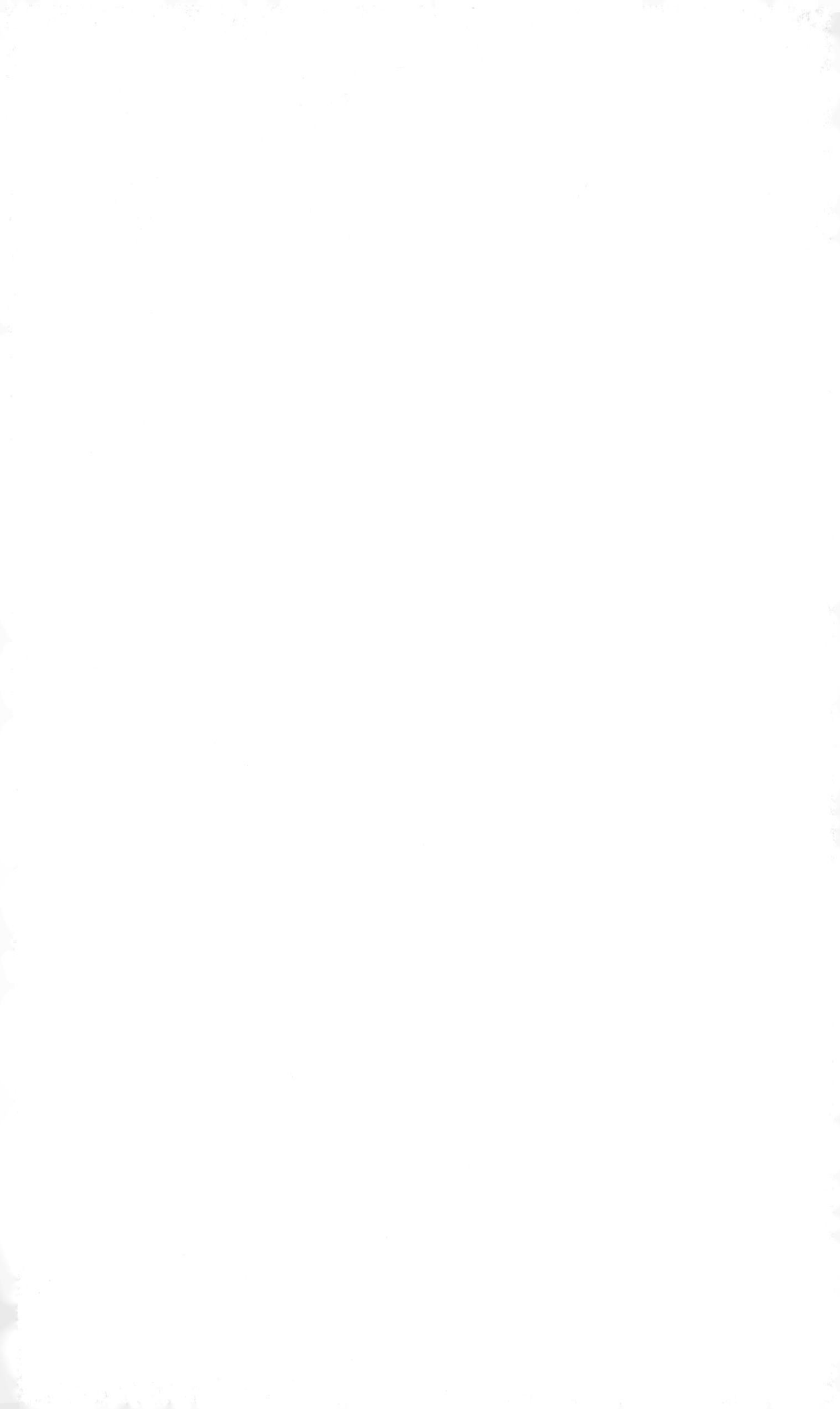

CPSIA information can be obtained
at www.ICGtesting.com
Printed in the USA
LVHW041517200519
618483LV00014B/1093/P